Alzheimer's
Transmission

Understanding the Prion Connection

Evelyn Kohl

Copyright

Table of Content

Overview of Alzheimer's Disease

Alzheimer's disease, named after Dr. Alois Alzheimer, who first diagnosed it in 1906, is a difficult challenge in the field of neurodegenerative illnesses. Alzheimer's disease is primarily characterised by increasing memory loss and cognitive deterioration, and it has a significant social and economic effect.

Pathophysiology

Alzheimer's disease is defined by two unique pathological features: the formation of amyloid-beta plaques and neurofibrillary tangles made up of tau protein.

These aberrant protein deposits impede neural connectivity, leading to neuronal death and brain shrinkage, notably in the hippocampus and cortex, which are critical for memory and cognition.

Symptoms and stages

Alzheimer's disease usually begins slowly, with moderate forgetfulness or confusion that is commonly mistaken for normal ageing symptoms.

As the illness develops, symptoms worsen, including severe memory loss, disorientation, changes in mood and behaviour, and difficulty with language and decision making. Alzheimer's disease is typically divided into three stages: early, medium, and late, which correspond to increasing levels of impairment.

Risk factors and genetics

While age remains the most important risk factor, with incidence growing significantly after 65, Alzheimer's is not an unavoidable component of ageing. Genetics, specifically the existence of the apolipoprotein E (APOE) ε4 allele, are highly connected with the condition.

However, it is crucial to highlight that genetic predisposition does not ensure illness development, meaning that environmental variables and lifestyle decisions may play a role.

Diagnoses and Management

Alzheimer's disease is diagnosed with a full clinical evaluation that includes a medical history review, neurological tests, and cognitive testing, which is often supplemented by imaging technologies such as MRI and PET scans.

While there is presently no cure, treatment options aim to alleviate symptoms and improve quality of life. These include pharmaceutical methods like cholinesterase inhibitors and NMDA receptor antagonists, as well as non-pharmacological therapy including cognitive stimulation and lifestyle changes.

Socioeconomic Impact

Alzheimer's has far-reaching consequences for families and carers, causing severe emotional and financial burden. From a social standpoint, the illness presents enormous issues, including increased healthcare expenditures, reduced productivity, and the need for long-term care facilities. Alzheimer's disease is predicted to become more common as the world's population ages, exacerbating these issues.

Emerging Research and Future Directions

Cutting-edge research is still being conducted to uncover the complexity of Alzheimer's disease, including the discovery of new treatment targets and diagnostic indicators.

Recent advances in understanding the disease's genetic and cellular underpinnings are opening up the possibility of disease-modifying medicines. Furthermore, there is increased interest in the impact of lifestyle factors and preventative treatments in lowering the risk of Alzheimer's, emphasising the significance of a comprehensive approach to this multidimensional disease.

To summarise, Alzheimer's disease is a multifaceted disorder that requires a thorough knowledge of its pathophysiology, risk factors, and social implications. Ongoing research and innovation are crucial in the search for effective therapies and, eventually, a cure, providing hope in the fight against this devastating illness.

Chapter 1: The concept of transmission in neurodegenerative disorders

Alzheimer's disease, Parkinson's disease, and Creutzfeldt-Jakob disease are examples of neurodegenerative illnesses, which are characterized by the gradual loss of neuronal structure and function. The notion of transmission is a relatively new and expanding topic of study in this subject, which investigates the potential that some characteristics of these disorders may be transmissible, similar to infectious diseases. This hypothesis substantially challenges our current understanding of neurodegenerative diseases.

Prion-like mechanisms

The concept of transmission in neurodegenerative illnesses gained popularity with the study of prions, infectious organisms that cause diseases such as Creutzfeldt-Jakob Disease.

Prions are misfolded proteins that may cause misfolding in other proteins, resulting in a cycle of misfolding and aggregation. This mechanism has prompted scientists to study if comparable mechanisms may be at work in other neurodegenerative illnesses.

Potential Transmission Pathways:

Proteins in Alzheimer's and Parkinson's disease, such as amyloid-beta and alpha-synuclein, have prion-like features, including the tendency to misfold and aggregate.

The idea proposes that these misfolded proteins might spread from cell to cell, and perhaps even between persons in certain conditions, but this is still being researched and debated.

Evidence from Clinical and Lab Studies

Several investigations have shown that symptoms of neurodegenerative disorders may occur near transplanted tissue, suggesting that the disease pathology may be transmitted.

Furthermore, experimental models have shown that the injection of misfolded proteins may cause disease in healthy brain areas, lending credence to the notion of a prion-like mechanism.

Iatrogenic Transmission

Concerns have also been raised concerning iatrogenic transmission, which occurs when the illness is mistakenly spread via medical procedures, especially in relation to growth hormone therapy and surgical tools. However, it is crucial to highlight that such occurrences are highly uncommon and have often included prion illnesses rather than more prevalent neurodegenerative conditions.

Implications in Public Health and Research

The idea of transmission in neurodegenerative illnesses has far-reaching ramifications. It requires a rethinking of how these illnesses are understood, diagnosed, and treated.

For example, if some neurodegenerative disorders can be transferred, although in very particular and rare conditions, it might have serious consequences for surgical operations, blood transfusions, and organ transplants.

Furthermore, knowing the transmission processes might lead to novel therapeutic options. If the distribution of misfolded proteins can be controlled or delayed, these illnesses' development may be slowed or stopped.

While the idea of transmission in neurodegenerative illnesses is still in its early stages and fraught with ambiguity, it marks a significant change in our understanding of these complicated diseases.

Ongoing research is critical in unravelling these riddles, since it has the potential to redefine disease processes while also leading to innovative treatment techniques and public health policies. As our knowledge grows, it becomes more important to exercise caution when using these principles in therapeutic contexts.

Chapter 2 : Understanding prions

Definition and Nature of Prions.

Prions are one of the most fascinating and mysterious creatures in the field of biological sciences. The word "prion" is derived from "proteinaceous infectious particle," and refers to a distinct form of pathogen made entirely of protein.

This section dives into the basic nature and properties of prions, offering insight on their involvement in illness and how they differ from other pathogens.

Basic Definition and Discovery

Stanley B. Prusiner proposed prions in the 1980s, a notion that was first regarded with scepticism but went on to win a Nobel Prize.

Prions, unlike typical pathogens like bacteria, viruses, and fungus, do not possess genetic material such as DNA or RNA. Instead, they are made up completely of improperly folded protein molecules.

Pathogenic Mechanism

The key protein implicated in prion illnesses is the prion protein (PrP), which is ordinarily present in a healthy form (PrP^C) in the body's cells. The pathogenic version of the prion protein, PrP^Sc, has a misfolded structure. Misfolded PrP^Sc interacts with normal PrP^C, causing it to convert into an aberrant form. This self-propagating process causes a buildup of misfolded proteins, which are harmful to brain cells.

Diseases caused by prions

Prion illnesses, commonly known as transmissible spongiform encephalopathies (TSEs), appear in a variety of forms in both animals and humans. Creutzfeldt-Jakob Disease (CJD) is the best-known human prion disease. Other variations include Gerstmann-Sträussler-Scheinker syndrome, fatal familial insomnia, and kuru.

In animals, prion diseases cause bovine spongiform encephalopathy (BSE, popularly known as "mad cow disease") in cattle, scrapie in sheep, and chronic wasting disease in deer and elk.

Prions have unique characteristics

Prions are distinctive for a number of reasons. For starters, they are very resistant to traditional sterilisation and disinfection procedures such as heat, radiation, and chemicals, making eradication especially difficult.

Second, they contradict the core dogma of molecular biology, which holds that genetic information flows from DNA to RNA to protein, by proving that proteins may convey infectious information even without genetic material.

Transmission and Incubation

Prion disorders may be transmitted by contaminated food, certain medical procedures, or, in certain circumstances, genetic mutations.

Prion illnesses are notorious for their extended incubation periods, which may span years or even decades before symptoms develop. Once symptoms appear, the illnesses usually advance quickly and are always deadly.

Public Health Concerns

The advent of BSE in the 1980s and its transmission to humans, resulting in variant Creutzfeldt-Jakob Disease (vCJD), demonstrated the ability of prions to traverse species boundaries. This prompted serious public health concerns and resulted in strict control measures in the food sector and healthcare facilities.

Understanding the biology of prions is critical not only for treating and preventing prion illnesses, but also for research into protein misfolding disorders.

The continued study of prions continues to challenge and improve our knowledge of infectious illnesses, molecular biology, and neurodegenerative processes, yielding exciting results that might have far-reaching ramifications in medical science.

Prions in Historical Context

The history of prions is both intriguing and complicated, charting their evolution from a cryptic disease agent to a well-defined clinical entity.

Early Observations and Theories

The history of prions starts with the discovery of scrapie, a disease affecting sheep and goats that has been known for generations. For a long time, the cause of scrapie was unknown.

Similar neurodegenerative illnesses in animals and humans, such as mad cow disease (BSE) and Creutzfeldt-Jakob disease (CJD), were discovered in the twentieth century, all of which had neuropathological parallels to scrapie.

Prusiner's groundbreaking work

Stanley Prusiner's breakthrough research in the 1980s revolutionised our knowledge of these disorders. He hypothesised that the causal culprit was a misfolded protein known as the prion, rather than a virus or bacteria.

Prusiner's prion theory was first viewed with scepticism since it questioned the widely held idea that nucleic acids were necessary for infection.

However, as evidence accumulated, his idea gained universal acceptance and was awarded the Nobel Prize in Physiology or Medicine in 1997.

The BSE crisis

The prion tale took a dramatic turn in the late twentieth century with the breakout of BSE in the United Kingdom. The outbreak, caused by feeding cattle meat-and-bone meal containing scrapie-infected sheep tissues, was catastrophic.

The later finding that BSE can be transferred to people, resulting in variant CJD, was a watershed moment in understanding prion diseases and their potential influence on public health.

How Prions Differentiate from Other Pathogens

Prions differ from other infections in three crucial ways:

Absence of nucleic acids

Unlike bacteria, viruses, and fungi, prions lack DNA and RNA. They are entirely protein-based, contradicting the widely held belief that genetic material is required for an agent to be infectious.

Mechanism of infection

Prions spread by causing misfolding in normal cellular prion proteins. This prion replication process, which relies on protein conformational changes rather than nucleic acid replication, is unusual among infectious pathogens.

Resistance to standard inactivation procedures.

Prions are very resistant to conventional techniques of sterilisation and inactivation, such as heat, radiation, and chemical treatments. The misfolded prion protein has a stable structure, which accounts for its durability.

Long incubation periods

Prion illnesses have extraordinarily extended incubation periods, which may last years or even decades. This prolonged latency period contrasts significantly with the comparatively quick development of symptoms after infection with other diseases.

Species Barriers and Adaptations

While prions may transcend species boundaries, as shown by the transmission of BSE to humans, the procedure is not simple.

The species barrier provides some protection, but once passed, prions may adapt to new hosts and possibly cause new disease types.

Invariably fatal outcomes

Prion disorders are presently incurable and usually lethal, causing severe neurodegeneration and death. This is in contrast to many viral or bacterial illnesses, which may be treated successfully.

Prions' evolutionary history and distinctive properties have had a profound influence on our knowledge of viral illnesses and neurodegeneration.

Prions have not only altered scholarly ideas on protein diseases, but they have also spurred significant modifications in public health policies, agricultural practices, and medical treatments throughout the globe.

As study proceeds, the tale of prions may provide even more breakthrough insights into the secrets of biology and illness.

Chapter 3: Alzheimer's Disease:A Closer look

Pathophysiology of Alzheimer's

Alzheimer's disease, a complicated and devastating neurodegenerative disorder, has a multiple pathophysiological mechanism. Understanding the process is critical for creating successful therapies and management methods.

Neuronal loss and brain atrophy

Alzheimer's is defined by the gradual loss of neurons and synapses in the brain, notably in the cortex and hippocampus, which are essential for memory and cognitive functioning. This neuronal degeneration causes considerable brain shrinkage and ventricular enlargement, which may be seen in the later stages of the illness.

Amyloid plaques

Amyloid-beta (Aβ) plaque formation is a critical characteristic in the pathophysiology of Alzheimer's disease. Aβ is a peptide derived from the cleavage of the amyloid precursor protein.

Alzheimer's disease is caused by faulty APP processing, resulting in Aβ buildup and insoluble plaques in the brain. These plaques are hypothesised to impede cell-to-cell communication and activate inflammatory responses, which contribute to neuronal injury.

Tau Tangles.

Another important feature of Alzheimer's disease is the growth of neurofibrillary tangles (NFTs) inside neurons. NFTs are made up of hyperphosphorylated tau, a protein that typically stabilises microtubules in neurons.

In Alzheimer's, aberrant tau creates twisted, insoluble fibres that impair the transport mechanism inside cells, causing cell death.

The Cholinergic Hypothesis

According to the cholinergic hypothesis, acetylcholine disruption plays a crucial role in Alzheimer's disease. Evidence of diminished cholinergic activity in Alzheimer's patients' brains lends credence to this notion, and several medications target this channel to relieve symptoms.

Genetic factors

While the vast majority of Alzheimer's cases are sporadic, genetic factors have an important influence, particularly in early-onset instances.

Mutations in genes such as APP, PSEN1, and PSEN2 are linked to familial Alzheimer's. The APOE ε4 allele is a recognised genetic risk factor for sporadic Alzheimer's, which affects amyloid deposition.

Inflammatory response and oxidative stress

Chronic inflammation and oxidative stress are also thought to contribute to Alzheimer's disease development. Neuroinflammation, caused by the immunological response to Aβ plaques and NFTs, worsens neuron damage.

Oxidative stress is caused by an imbalance between reactive oxygen species and the body's capacity to detoxify them, which leads to neurodegeneration.

Vascular Contributions

New study reveals that vascular variables, such as decreased blood flow and blood-brain barrier integrity, may contribute to Alzheimer's development and progression. These conditions may aggravate amyloid deposition and neuronal loss.

Alzheimer's disease pathogenesis is complicated, with several interacting pathways. These include amyloid and tau pathology, cholinergic dysfunction, hereditary variables, inflammatory responses, oxidative stress, and vascular components.

Understanding these pathways is critical for developing targeted medicines and eventually changing the course of this dreadful illness. As research progresses, new insights into the mechanism of Alzheimer's disease emerge, providing hope for more effective future treatments.

Symptoms and Progressions

Alzheimer's disease shows as a slow development of symptoms that may be divided into three stages: early, medium, and late, each with its own set of obstacles.

Early Stage (mild Alzheimer's)

Symptoms in the early stages are frequently mild and might be mistaken for age-related changes or stress. They include:

- Memory gaps occur, particularly when remembering recent events or discussions.

- Difficulty with complicated duties and planning, such as financial management.

- Changes in personality and mood, such as despair or indifference.

- Minor confusion, such as losing track of the date or time of day.

Middle Stage (moderate Alzheimer's)
As the illness advances into the middle stage, symptoms worsen and interfere with everyday activities. This includes:

- Increased memory loss and disorientation, including forgetting personal history and failing to recognise friends and relatives.
- Difficulties with language, such as finding the appropriate words.

- Behavioural changes, such as wandering, agitation, or improper behaviour.

- Routine actions, such as dressing or bathing, provide challenges.

Late stage (severe Alzheimer's)

Individuals in their latter phases demand full-time care. Symptoms include:

- Individuals often struggle to speak effectively due to severe memory loss.

- Physical challenges include walking, sitting, and, ultimately, swallowing.

- Increased susceptibility to infections, especially pneumonia.

- Complete reliance on carers for everyday tasks.

Diagnosis and Treatment Options

Diagnosis

There is no one test for Alzheimer's disease, thus diagnosing it requires a mix of tests. The method involves:

- Medical history and symptom evaluation.
- Cognitive and neuropsychological exams are used to assess memory, problem-solving, attention, counting, and language skills.

- Brain imaging (MRI or CT scans) is used to rule out alternative causes of dementia and monitor brain changes.

- Blood tests are used to rule out other illnesses that may cause symptoms similar to Alzheimer's.

Treatment Options:

While there is no cure for Alzheimer's, existing therapies are designed to alleviate symptoms and enhance quality of life.

Pharmaceutical treatments

- Cholinesterase inhibitors (including donepezil, rivastigmine, and galantamine) are used to treat mild to severe Alzheimer's disease. They function by raising the levels of acetylcholine, a neurotransmitter linked to memory and learning.

- Memantine, which treats moderate to severe Alzheimer's, works by controlling glutamate, another crucial brain chemical involved in learning and memory.

Non-pharmacological approaches.

- Cognitive stimulation and activities customised to the individual's ability may aid in maintaining cognitive function.

- Lifestyle improvements, such as frequent exercise, a nutritious diet, and social interaction, are helpful.

- Behavioural tactics for treating symptoms such as agitation or sleep difficulties.

Supportive Care

As Alzheimer's disease worsens, providing supportive care becomes more important.

This involves creating a safe living environment, assisting with everyday tasks, and managing medical difficulties.

Future and Experimental Therapeutics

Ongoing research is looking at novel therapeutic options, including as pharmaceuticals targeting amyloid and tau proteins, immunotherapy, and lifestyle changes to halt disease development.

Chapter 4: The Connection between Alzheimer's disease and Prion

Exploring the Link

The putative link between Alzheimer's disease and prions has sparked considerable scholarly attention. This investigation is based on the parallels identified in the protein misfolding and aggregation mechanisms that are common to both diseases.

Understanding Protein Misfolding

Misfolded proteins, such as amyloid-beta (Aβ) and tau, in Alzheimer's disease cause plaques and tangles that harm neurons. Similarly, prion illnesses entail the misfolding of the prion protein (PrP), which leads to a cascade of neurodegeneration. The similarities between these pathways raise the possibility that Alzheimer's disease has prion-like features.

Research findings

Several research have looked at this connection. Key findings include:

The capacity of amyloid-beta and tau to cause misfolding in healthy proteins, similar to prions, suggests a prion-like mode of dissemination.

Experiments have shown that injecting Alzheimer's brain extracts into animal models may cause Alzheimer-like pathology, suggesting a possibility for transmission similar to prion diseases.

Transmission Studies

The issue of Alzheimer's being "transmissible" has mostly been investigated in terms of medical operations. For example, in the past, patients who got growth hormone produced from human cadavers had unexpectedly high levels of amyloid pathology, suggesting that amyloid seeds might be transmitted. However, these occurrences are highly uncommon and entail very particular conditions.

Differences from Classic Prion Diseases

Despite these similarities, it is critical to separate Alzheimer's from classic prion disorders such as Creutzfeldt-Jakob Disease. Alzheimer's does not have the same contagious properties as CJD or other prion illnesses.

The transfer of Alzheimer's pathology has not been demonstrated in natural settings, and the illness is not considered infectious in the traditional sense.

Implications in Treatment and Research

Understanding if and how Alzheimer's disease and prion illnesses share pathways might have substantial implications for therapy development. If Alzheimer's disease spreads by a prion-like mechanism, addressing this process might provide new treatment options.

Furthermore, this relationship necessitates a reevaluation of safety standards in surgical and medical settings in order to reduce any conceivable danger of transmission, no matter how theoretical.

While the theory that Alzheimer's disease has prion-like features is attractive, it is still being researched and debated. The parallels between protein misfolding and aggregation provide exciting opportunities for understanding Alzheimer's disease and generating new therapies.

However, the difference between Alzheimer's and infectious prion illnesses remains evident in terms of contagion and transmission. Further study is required to fully understand the intricacies of these neurodegenerative processes and their possible relationships.

Case Studies & Clinical Evidence

The examination of the suspected prion-like properties of Alzheimer's disease covers a variety of case studies and clinical data, giving insights into this complicated and fascinating element of neurodegenerative disease research.

Case Studies for Iatrogenic Transmission

Case studies involving patients who received cadaver-derived human growth hormone (hGH) or dura mater transplants provide a considerable amount of data.

Post-mortem studies of several individuals decades after the treatment showed unexpected amyloid-beta (Aβ) pathology, akin to Alzheimer's disease, despite the lack of clinical symptoms throughout their lives.

These results prompted concerns regarding the iatrogenic spread of amyloid disease.

Neuropathological Findings in Brain Transplant Recipients

Another fascinating collection of case studies concerns people who have had neuronal tissue transplants from foetal origins.

In other individuals who died from other reasons, post-mortem examinations revealed that the transplanted tissue acquired Alzheimer's-like pathology, including amyloid plaques and tau tangles. This raises the prospect of a "seed" effect, in which misfolded proteins from the recipient's brain cause disease in transplanted tissue.

Amyloid-beta transmission in animal models

Experimental research have been critical in determining this link. Researchers discovered that putting brain extracts from Alzheimer's patients into animal models causes Alzheimer's-like amyloid pathology in the animals.

These findings provide credence to the notion that a transmissible factor exists in Alzheimer's pathogenesis, at least under certain experimental settings.

Clinical Evidence for Familial Alzheimer's Disease

Familial Alzheimer's disease, caused by mutations in certain genes, offers a unique view of the illness's evolution. Because this kind of Alzheimer's is predictable, early pathological alterations may be studied, providing insight into the potential function of protein misfolding and aggregation in disease development and progression.

Epidemiological Data

While there is no clear epidemiological proof that Alzheimer's is infectious in the general population, research in this subject provides insights into disease propagation patterns inside the brain as well as possible risk factors for disease development.

Research on Neurosurgical Instruments

Some investigations have looked into the possible possibility of Alzheimer's disease spread via neurosurgical tools. While prions are known to stick to surgical steel and withstand routine sterilisation methods, there is presently no clear proof that surgical equipment have spread Alzheimer's disease.

Implications for Public Health and Medical Practice

The case studies and clinical data presented so far highlight the need of exercising care when assessing the probable transmissibility of Alzheimer's disease. While evidence shows a prion-like mechanism in Alzheimer's pathology, this does not mean that the illness is contagious in the same way as classic prion diseases are.

However, these discoveries have spurred a reconsideration of medical procedures, notably in terms of surgical equipment sterilisation and brain tissue management.

To summarise, case studies and clinical data contribute to a more sophisticated understanding of Alzheimer's disease's possible prion-like features. While these results are intriguing and have important implications for research and medical practice, they must be viewed within the larger framework of Alzheimer's research. Continued research is required to fully understand the intricacies of Alzheimer's disease and its probable progression pathways.

Chapter 5: Transmission Pathways

Known and Theoretical Transmission Routes

The investigation of transmission channels in Alzheimer's disease entails differentiating between recognised routes in classical prion illnesses and speculative, but unconfirmed, routes in Alzheimer's.

Understanding these routes is critical for determining the dangers to public health and medical operations.

Classical Prion Disease Transmission

Classical prion illnesses, such as Creutzfeldt-Jakob disease (CJD), have known transmission channels that include

Iatrogenic Transmission: Historically, prion disorders have been transferred by medical procedures such as human growth hormone injections and corneal transplants from contaminated donors.

Oral Ingestion: The epidemic of Bovine Spongiform Encephalopathy (BSE), sometimes known as "mad cow disease," emphasised oral ingestion as a method via which animals swallowed prion-contaminated feed, resulting in transmission to humans.

Familial Transmission: Some prion disorders are caused by inherited genetic mutations, resulting in familial transmission.

Theoretical Transmission of Alzheimer's

Alzheimer's disease transmission is a theoretical idea that has not been confirmed in natural human-to-human or animal-to-human encounters. Possible theoretical approaches include:

Iatrogenic Transmission: As with prions, there is a potential possibility of transferring Alzheimer's pathology via medical procedures that involve brain tissue, such as neurosurgery, albeit no documented instances exist.

Transplantation and Blood Transfusion: In theory, organ or tissue transplantation from Alzheimer's patients, as well as blood transfusions, might be used to transfer harmful proteins. However, there is no definite proof for this in Alzheimer's disease.

Cell-to-Cell move Within the Brain: While not a direct transmission pathway, Alzheimer's pathology is hypothesised to move from cell to cell within the brain in a prion-like fashion. This intracerebral spread is an important area of study for understanding the disease's course.

Controversial and unproven Hypotheses

Certain theories propose more problematic approaches, such as:

Environmental Exposure: The concept of environmental variables having a role in Alzheimer's disease, maybe via misfolded proteins, is theoretical, with no strong proof.

Infectious Agents: There are ideas that infectious agents, such as viruses or bacteria, may play a role in Alzheimer's pathogenesis. However, these hypotheses need more scientific support.

In conclusion, although conventional prion illnesses have well-established transmission pathways, the idea of transmission in Alzheimer's disease is primarily theoretical and hypothetical. Current research does not support the assumption that Alzheimer's is an infectious illness in the traditional sense. Ongoing research into the processes of protein misfolding and aggregation in Alzheimer's is critical to better understanding these pathways and their implications for disease treatment and public health strategies.

Investigating Iatrogenic Transmission.

Iatrogenic transmission is the accidental spread of a disease as a consequence of medical operations or therapy. In the context of Alzheimer's disease, determining this possible pathway is critical for patient safety.

Historical Cases and Concerns

The principal worry stemmed from previous incidences of Creutzfeldt-Jakob condition (CJD), in which individuals got the condition after undergoing treatments such as human growth hormone therapy or dura mater transplants from cadavers.

These cases raised worries regarding the possibility of iatrogenic Alzheimer's transmission, especially considering amyloid-beta proteins' prion-like characteristics.

Research and Findings

Research exploring the likelihood of Alzheimer's transmission via surgical equipment or tissue transplants has been mainly inconclusive, although it remains an area of research. No direct evidence has been discovered to support such transmission in clinical settings.

Studies have looked at how amyloid-beta proteins attach to surgical tools and how resistant they are to regular sterilisation techniques. While these investigations suggest a theoretical danger, the actual risk in clinical practice seems to be minimal.

Current Guidelines and Practices

In response to these concerns, medical rules and practices have been revised to incorporate more stringent sterilisation protocols, particularly in neurosurgery and operations affecting the central nervous system.

To reduce possible risks, synthetic or properly tested biological materials have been recommended for grafts and transplants.

Environmental and Genetic Susceptibility

The interaction of environmental and genetic susceptibility is an important topic of study in understanding the risk and progression of Alzheimer's disease.

Genetic Susceptibility

The APOE ε4 allele, among other genetic variables, dramatically increases the risk of Alzheimer's disease. However, having these genes does not ensure illness development, suggesting that environmental variables play an important role.

Familial Alzheimer's disease, caused by mutations in genes such as APP, PSEN1, and PSEN2, accounts for a tiny proportion of cases but sheds light on the genetic pathways underlying the illness.

Environmental influences

Lifestyle variables such as food, exercise, and cognitive engagement have been proven to impact Alzheimer's risk. A heart-healthy lifestyle, for example, seems to reduce the risk.

Exposure to some environmental toxins, such as heavy metals or air pollution, has been considered as a risk factor, although no strong causative links have been proven.

Gene-Environment Interactions

The relationship between genetic predisposition and environmental influences is complicated. Individuals with genetic risk factors may be more vulnerable to environmental impacts, while certain behaviours may reduce hereditary risks.

This research seeks to understand how these interactions contribute to the development and progression of Alzheimer's disease, with the goal of developing more personalised preventive and treatment techniques.

A thorough knowledge of Alzheimer's disease requires an investigation of both iatrogenic transmission and the combination of environmental variables and genetic predisposition. While the potential of iatrogenic transmission is primarily theoretical, it highlights the need of strict medical standards. Understanding the intricate interaction between genes and the environment might lead to more targeted therapies and preventative measures, thereby lowering the prevalence and effect of Alzheimer's disease.

Chapter 6:Public Health Implications

Impact on Healthcare Policies

The public health implications of Alzheimer's disease, especially given its probable prion-like properties, have a substantial influence on healthcare policy.

Revising Sterilisation and Surgical Procedures.

Policies may need to be amended to incorporate improved sterilisation measures for surgical tools, particularly in neurosurgery, to reduce the danger of spreading proteinopathies.

Screening & Monitoring

Healthcare policy might include more stringent screening and monitoring techniques for neurodegenerative illnesses, particularly in populations with recognised risk factors.

Resource Allocation

As the incidence of Alzheimer's disease rises, healthcare systems must address the allocation of resources for research, treatment, and carer support.

Public Awareness and Education

Policies should prioritise public education regarding Alzheimer's, including symptoms, progression, and the need of early detection.

Ethical and Social Considerations

Alzheimer's illness has far-reaching ethical and societal ramifications.

Stigma and Discrimination.
Addressing the stigma associated with Alzheimer's is critical. Public education efforts may increase knowledge of the condition while lowering fear and prejudice.

Decision Making and Autonomy
Ethical concerns emerge about the autonomy and decision-making abilities of Alzheimer's patients, especially those in severe stages. Policies must guarantee that their rights and dignity are protected.

Carer Support

The load on carers is immense. Ethical issues include giving enough assistance and resources to carers for Alzheimer's patients.

Genetic Tests and Privacy

With the significance of genetics in Alzheimer's, ethical concerns about genetic testing and privacy arise. Policies must strike a balance between the advantages of genetic information and the right to privacy and informed consent.

Strategies for Prevention and Control

Alzheimer's disease prevention and control strategies are key components of public health planning.

Lifestyle Modifications

Promoting heart-healthy behaviours such as a balanced diet, frequent exercise, and cognitive engagement may lower the chance of acquiring Alzheimer's.

Early diagnosis and intervention

Improving techniques of early identification and intervention may help to decrease disease development. Cognitive screening and early treatment alternatives should be made available as part of public health measures.

Research & Development

Investing in research to better understand, treat, and prevent Alzheimer's disease is critical. This includes funding for research into its possible prion-like features and associated ramifications.

Community-Based Care.

Creating community-based care choices may help Alzheimer's patients and their families while lessening the strain on hospital systems.

International Collaboration

Alzheimer's disease is a worldwide concern. Effective preventive and control measures rely heavily on international cooperation in research, policymaking, and best practice exchange.

Alzheimer's disease has significant public health consequences, necessitating comprehensive interventions that include healthcare policy changes, ethical concerns, and a multifaceted approach to prevention and control. These initiatives involve cross-sector cooperation, continuing research, and a commitment to meeting the needs of both Alzheimer's patients and carers.

Innovative Research on Alzheimer's and Prions

Recent developments in Alzheimer's and prion research have provided fresh insights and paved the road for future treatments.

Targeting Protein Misfolding and Aggregation.

One of the most promising areas of study is avoiding the misfolding and aggregation of proteins such as amyloid-beta and tau in Alzheimer's and PrP in prion disorders. Novel chemicals and immunotherapies are being developed to target these proteins and prevent harmful buildup.

Gene Therapy and CRISPR Technology

Gene therapy and CRISPR-Cas9 technologies provide novel approaches to Alzheimer's treatment, especially in situations where the disease is genetically based. Researchers use gene editing to fix mutations or regulate gene expression in order to avoid illness development or progression.

Biomarker Development

The creation of biomarkers for early detection is critical. Neuroimaging advances and the discovery of biochemical markers in blood or cerebrospinal fluid show promise.

These indicators may help detect Alzheimer's and prion illnesses at an early stage, even before symptoms develop.

Understanding the Prion-like Mechanisms in Alzheimer's

Researchers are increasingly interested in understanding how prion-like pathways may contribute to Alzheimer's disease. This involves investigating the transfer of misfolded proteins throughout the brain and their possible involvement in disease progression.

Neuroinflammation and Immune System

The function of neuroinflammation and the immune system in Alzheimer's and prion disorders is an emerging field of study. To delay or prevent neurodegeneration, researchers are looking into creating medicines that target inflammatory pathways or control the immune response.

Stem Cell Research

Stem cell research has the potential to help understand disease causes and find novel therapies. Researchers may examine Alzheimer's cellular mechanisms and test novel treatments by growing neurons from patient-derived stem cells.

AI and Big Data

The application of artificial intelligence and big data is changing Alzheimer's research. AI systems can analyse massive volumes of medical data to detect trends, forecast illness development, and tailor treatment plans.

Alzheimer's and prions research is fast advancing, with new findings providing promise for improved diagnosis, treatment, and, perhaps, prevention of these terrible illnesses. As our knowledge grows, the future avenues of this study show significant potential for changing the face of neurodegenerative disease therapy and management.

Potential Therapeutic Approaches.

Recent advances in Alzheimer's research have revealed numerous prospective therapy options aimed at halting or slowing disease development or alleviating symptoms.

Disease-modifying Therapies

Disease-modifying medications are being developed to address the fundamental causes of Alzheimer's, such as the buildup of amyloid-beta and tau proteins. These include monoclonal antibodies targeted to remove these proteins from the brain.

Neuroprotective strategies

Neuroprotective medicines are being investigated as potential treatments for Alzheimer's disease. This comprises antioxidants and anti-inflammatory compounds.

Tau-targeting therapies

Given the importance of tau in Alzheimer's, treatments targeting tau pathology are being investigated. These include tau aggregation inhibitors and immunotherapies that reduce tau tangles.

Cognitive enhancers

Current medications, such as cholinesterase inhibitors and memantine, that attempt to enhance cognitive function and decrease cognitive decline, are being developed and coupled with other medicines to increase effectiveness.

Lifestyle Interventions and Brain Health Programmes

Non-pharmacological treatments, such as nutrition, exercise, cognitive training, and social interaction, are being promoted for their ability to prevent the development or progression of Alzheimer's.

Stem cell therapy

Stem cell treatment is an active research topic with the potential to regenerate or repair damaged brain tissue, albeit this technique is currently primarily experimental.

Forecasts and Emerging Trends

The area of Alzheimer's research is dynamic, with various forecasts and new trends influencing its future direction.

Personalised Medicine

Advances in genetics and biomarkers are opening the way for personalised medicine approaches in Alzheimer's, where therapies may be customised to individual genetic profiles and disease pathways.

Concentrate on prevention

There is a rising emphasis on preventative techniques, such as identifying and addressing risk factors early in life, before symptoms appear.

Combination Therapies

Recognising Alzheimer's multifaceted character, combination treatments that target various elements of the illness at once are likely to gain popularity.

Artificial Intelligence for Drug Discovery

AI and machine learning are rapidly being used to discover novel drug targets, forecast disease development, and tailor therapy approaches.

Global Collaboration and Data Sharing

The complexities of Alzheimer's research need international cooperation and data exchange. Large-scale multinational collaborations and consortiums are becoming increasingly prevalent, hastening the speed of discovery.

Conclusion

Summary of Key Insights

The study of Alzheimer's disease and its possible link to prions has provided vital insights into the genesis and course of neurodegenerative illnesses. Key findings include:

Alzheimer's is a complicated illness that includes amyloid-beta plaques, tau tangles, neuronal death, and cognitive impairment.

Prion-like processes: Studies show that Alzheimer's disease may include prion-like processes in which misfolded proteins spread throughout the brain, leading to the illness's development.

Potential Transmission Routes: While the theoretical potential of transmission, especially iatrogenic, has been investigated, Alzheimer's disease is not considered infectious in the same way as classical prion illnesses are.

Advances in Treatment: Current treatments concentrate on symptom management, but new medicines seek to address the underlying illness processes.

Future Research Needs

To increase our knowledge and treatment of Alzheimer's, future research requirements include:

Elucidating Prion-like features: Further study into Alzheimer's prion-like features is critical for better understanding disease progression and developing novel therapies.

Biomarker Development: Finding accurate biomarkers for Alzheimer's disease diagnosis and surveillance will be crucial.

Therapeutic Innovation: Researchers should concentrate on creating disease-modifying medicines, such as those targeting amyloid-beta and tau pathologies.

Preventive techniques: More research on lifestyle interventions and risk factor modification is required to create effective preventive techniques.

Genetic and Environmental Interactions: Understanding the relationship between genetic susceptibility and environmental variables will aid in the development of personalised therapies.

Conclusion on Alzheimer's and Prions

The route of understanding Alzheimer's and its possible link to prions exemplifies the complexities and difficulty of comprehending neurodegenerative illnesses.

The interesting notion that Alzheimer's and prion illnesses share pathways offers up new study and therapeutic opportunities. While Alzheimer's disease remains a serious medical and societal problem, ongoing advances in science, driven by innovation and multidisciplinary cooperation, provide hope.

As we get a better knowledge of these illnesses, we will be able to develop more effective management, treatment, and preventive measures for Alzheimer's disease and associated neurodegenerative disorders. The road is as difficult as it is promising, yet each new discovery puts us one step closer to solving the riddles of these complicated illnesses.